# FAITH & ILLNESS

## REFLECTIONS ON GOD'S
## SUSTAINING LOVE

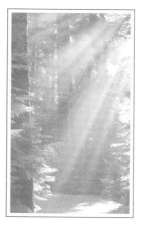

by Nancy Groves

Published by
Patient Press
6475 Perimeter Drive, P. O. Box 110, Dublin, Ohio 43016 U.S.A.

Library of Congress Cataloging-in-Publication Data
Groves, Nancy.
    Faith & illness : reflections on God's sustaining
  love / by Nancy Groves. -- 1st ed.

      p. cm.
      LCCN 2001094361
      ISBN 0-9701545-3-4
    1. Sick--Religious life.   2. Christian life.
  3. Adjustment (Psychology)   I. Title.

BL625.9.S53G76 2002     291.4'42
                        QBI01-701077

Cover design and book production by Ruth Marcus, Sequim, WA
Cover photograph by Ross Hamilton, Sequim, WA

IN MEMORY OF

Don Groves
whose spirit of love
remains with us forever.


DEDICATED TO

Katherine Groves
whose life embraces
her father's joy.

# CONTENTS

I    Introduction   vii

II    Something's Wrong—
Searching for an Answer   1

III    What am I Feeling?   9
         Shock   11
         Anxiety   19
         Anger   27
         Depression   35
         Guilt   45
         Shame   53

IV    Adjusting to Endless Changes   59

V    Survival   81

VI    Healing   91

VII    Peace   105

VIII    God's Gift of Healing   111

IX    About the Publisher   121

# INTRODUCTION

The crisis of ill health affects us all
at some time in our lives.
For many of us, the duration is short,
and recovery is soon.

However, there are others who must
confront the crisis of a chronic
progressive disease, or a life
threatening illness, and this
reality may be a continuing part of life.

The onset of the disease may be
at any age, making the road
ahead one filled with fears,
apprehensions,
and anxieties.

Too often, that road is traveled alone.

If you are on this road, then this book hopes to be your companion —

- to be a guide to understanding the emotional impact of facing a serious illness,

- to provide comfort for the days when your heart is weary from the struggle,

- to heighten your awareness to your uniqueness and beauty that no disease can touch or change,

- to remind you of God's sustaining compassion and His everlasting love.

# SOMETHING'S WRONG

## SEARCHING FOR AN ANSWER

I will trust and not be afraid;
for the Lord God is my strength
and my song, and he has become
my salvation.

*Isaiah  12:2*

How many days or months have
passed with the recurring
feelings of fatigue and discomfort,
and of having a sense that all is
not right within?

The internal messages are
constant, yet subtle,
reminding me of storm clouds
ominously forming in the skies.

I am left to wonder when
the storm
   will
      appear.

I feel helpless and
frightened.

My doctor is concerned.
His face mirrors my
apprehensions. He
cannot diagnose the
problem until more tests
are done. I am tired of
subjecting my body
to the invasions of strange
tubes and x-rays.

I am becoming an illness
to be diagnosed instead
of a person who is
suffering.

See me.
  SEE ME PLEASE.

It is over. The illness
has been named. I am
part of a national
average — a statistic —
and I am sometimes
referred to as my disease.

That only increases my pain.

It is over.
    The illness has been named.

It is over —
    or is this only the
        beginning for
            me?

**REFLECTIONS**

Knowing the disease I must face brings new concerns to me. What do I need to know about my illness?

Has the knowledge of this illness changed my priorities in life?

What is most important to me now?

## DEVOTIONS

Dear God,

I am frightened. I wanted an
answer. Now I have received one,
and I am afraid. I want this to be
a bad dream that will end when I
awaken to tomorrow's sunlight.
But tomorrow's arrival will not
erase the reality of today.

Stay close, dear God, and
let me feel the warmth of your
Son's light on me as I face today…
and tomorrow.

Amen

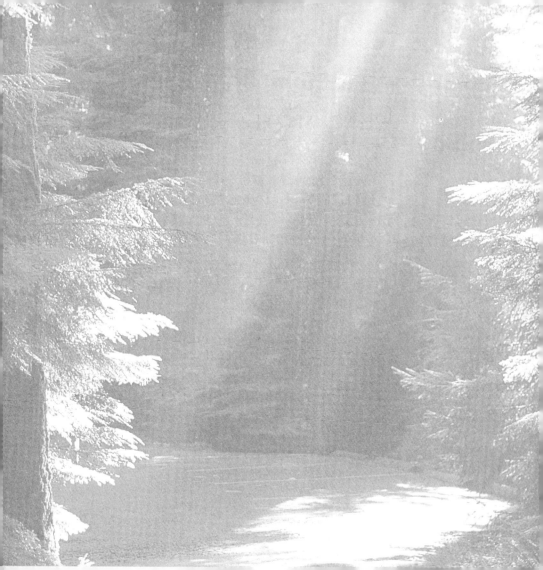

# WHAT AM I FEELING?

SHOCK
ANXIETY
ANGER
DEPRESSION
GUILT
SHAME

**Let not your hearts be troubled,
neither let them be afraid.**

*John 14:27*

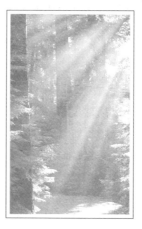

**Trust in Him at all times . . .
pour out your heart before
Him; God is a refuge for us.**

*Psalms 62:8*


Sad
Hurt
Outraged
Confused
broKen

I know now what I must face.
The cause of my apprehensions
has been named. But the future
is still filled with unknowns.
The uncertainties frighten me.

What am I feeling?

What makes that question
so difficult to answer?

It is as though my body
were not my own, as though
a stranger had invaded my
frame. I feel cut off from
my emotions.

I am numb, overwhelmed,
afraid I will be unable to
cope. I can't face it –
not yet. I don't want to
discuss it, for then it
becomes too real
for me.

I want life to continue
on as before. Talk with
me about the news, the
weather, the latest fashions,
anything but sickness.

Don't look at me with
sadness in your eyes,
or sympathy,
        or fear.
That only shows me the
pain I have brought to
you. I can't deal with
that now.

I need some distance
from this new reality.

Let me find comfort
in ignoring this —
in denying this —
if I must.

Denial is my refuge.

Allow me that.

**REFLECTIONS**

What was my immediate reaction to the news of my illness?

How did that reaction help me to cope with this news?

## REFLECTIONS

What is my reaction to my illness now?
How is it different?

What have I learned about myself?

## DEVOTIONS

Dear God,

I thought I was strong, but
I am not. I thought I could face
this, but I cannot. I thought I
could handle anything — I
was wrong. Instead, I hide, but
I cannot hide from you, dear
God. You have always been
with me. Your presence enters
my thoughts and my heart. The
strength of your love sustains me
in the midst of this inner turmoil.
You are my refuge.

Amen.

**Cast all your anxieties on
Him, for He cares about you.**

*I Peter 5:7*


**A**pprehensive
**N**ervous
e**X**hausted
**I**nsecure
**E**mpty
**T**ense
uneas**Y**

Feelings of apprehension
are beginning to surface.
At times, the anxiety seems
immobilizing.

How can I unlock its grip?

Perhaps I need to examine
these feelings more closely.
I ask myself...

What brings this anxiety?

Just asking the question
frees me to discover
the answer.

The source is fear.

I am afraid of the
uncertainties that lie ahead.

I am afraid of loneliness —
afraid that my illness will
keep others away.

I am afraid of the pain
and sorrow I may have
to endure.

I am afraid
    of losing control,
    of losing my abilities,
    of losing parts of my body,
            of losing myself.

My awareness of these fears
lessens the anxiety for me.
It does not remove the
anxiety from my life, but it
seems to make it less
overwhelming and more
manageable.

I have learned that being
afraid is okay. I realize there
is a purpose to my fears.
They give me opportunities
to grow beyond them.

Sharing my fears is the
next step for me.
Keeping them within
brings emotional isolation
and depression.

Finding someone to listen
may not be easy. I know
my illness can trigger many
fears in others, making
avoidance easier for them.

But I must approach
others and invite them
into my life. I must take
care of myself and teach
others what I need
from them.

Those
who are open to me,
who love me, and
who are willing to learn
will take away the fears
and be my refuge
in this time of need.

How precious they
are to me.

## REFLECTIONS

What fears am I experiencing as a result
of this illness?

Are these fears helping me?

What would lessen these fears for me?

## DEVOTIONS

Dear God,

There is a comfort in bringing my fears to you, for I know that your love is greater than all the anxieties of this world. I hear your gentle wisdom in the words of my loved ones who respond to my apprehensions. I call to you, and your voice brings me to a place of tranquility once again. Thank you for loving me.

Amen.

**Cast your burden on the Lord,
and he will sustain you.**

*Psalms 55:22*

Annoyed
eNraged
Guilty
Exasperated
Regretful

These last few days have been
increasingly difficult for me.
I seem to lash out at others for
no apparent reason.

I am negative and sarcastic
to people who are trying to
be kind and understanding.

What is going on within me?

I am told I seem angry. Can
I admit to feeling angry?

Anger isn't always
understood or accepted.
It usually scares people
away and causes others
to be critical and judgmental.

And yet,
      I AM ANGRY.

I am angry that I have been
afflicted with this illness.

I am angry that I must be
dependent on others.

I am angry that I have
been relieved of responsibilities
that I am still able to assume.

I am angry that people
treat me differently now.

I am angry that I am
losing control over my
life.

I AM ANGRY
        and
I feel guilty because
        of my anger.

It is okay to be angry —

        I am human.

Since my bed is oftentimes
my only companion in
the day, I have learned to
leave my anger there.

Beating the pillows is a
favorite pastime for me.
It is harmless to others and
allows me to get rid of the
anger that would otherwise
keep loved ones away.

Sharing my anger with God
gives me a listener who
accepts me where
I am and who
tells me . . .
> He can handle it.

Yes,
> I am angry
>> and
> I accept where I am
>> and
> I can handle it...now.

IT IS OKAY TO BE ANGRY...
> I AM HUMAN.

**REFLECTIONS**

How do I show my anger?

Can I accept anger as being a normal and understandable reaction to my illness?

What helps me to get rid of my anger?

## DEVOTIONS

Dear God,

As a child of God, I worry about
my anger, for this feeling contradicts
many of your teachings. And yet, to deny
my anger would only add to the
difficulties I am facing. My intent is
not to harm anyone in my life. The
anger comes from a different place…
it masks my fears. Sometimes, it is
easier to be angry than to be afraid.
So I bring my anger to you, knowing
that your loving arms will lift this
burden, embrace me, and bring
me comfort.

Amen.

**Surely He has borne our griefs and carried our sorrows.**

*Isaiah 53:4*

Despondent
Empty
Powerless
Regretful
Exasperated
Sorrowful
Solemn
Isolated
Overwhelmed
Numb

I don't think I can face today.

I have no energy to leave this
bed or to talk with anyone.
I seem to be in a place
I've not been before.

I feel hopeless.

There seems to be no
reason to continue with
my life. I can't control
my tears. They are endless
as they stream down my face
and fall into my empty hands.

Isn't my life also empty —
void of meaning and
purpose?

I have lost my valiant
fight with this illness.

I have no strength to go on.

My loved ones seem
frightened of my sorrow.
They bring me gifts, shower
me with flowers to
        "cheer me up."

They are constantly
doing something
for me...

> straightening my
> > sheets
> fluffing my
> > pillows
> opening my
> > drapes
> reading my
> > get well cards
> bringing my
> > food.

I wonder if they are doing
these things to avoid the
emotional discomfort my
illness brings.

Their acts of kindness
do not go unnoticed,
although I am unable to
convey any appreciation.

The sorrow and the
emptiness remain.

In the midst of these
caring people, scurrying
to do something to lift
my spirits, I feel
    isolated
        and
            alone.

I feel no comfort.

Then you enter my room.
You see my tears.
My sadness frightens
you. Your face searches
mine for an answer...

I have none to give you.

You draw near to me, place
your arms around me, and I
rest my head upon your shoulder.
I hold you close. My tears fall.
We do not speak. And yet, your
presence tells me of your love
and compassion.

Your gift to me is
yourself, your
honest,
　　silent and beautiful
　　　　expression of
　　　　　　compassion.

Your gift of presence
relieves my feelings
of isolation and despair.

While others are
*doing* for me,
　　you are
　　　　*being* with me.

That is what I need right now.
That is what comforts my soul.

Thank you
   for being in my life.

Today, you shared my
pain and sadness.

Tomorrow will be a better day.

I think I can face
   tomorrow
      all because
         of you.

## REFLECTIONS

What makes this illness most difficult for me?

What comforts me when I feel hopeless and
in despair?

How can I receive what I need from others?

## DEVOTIONS

Dear God,

The sadness I am feeling extends
beyond my physical body and touches
my soul. I feel so distant from your
love…so alone with this illness.
I have cried out to you in my prayers,
asking for a sign of your presence.
And you answered in the form of
a beloved friend whose physical
embrace carried your love to
my soul.

Amen.

**Let him return to the Lord, that
He may have mercy on him,
and to our God, for He will
abundantly pardon.**

*Isaiah 55:7*

Grieved
Upset
Inadequate
Loathsome
Troubled

I need to find a reason for this illness.

I ask myself
  over and
    over again,
      Why Me?

In my search for an answer,
I remember past behaviors
that…
  may have offended
  may have caused pain
  may have been unjust
      uncalled for
      egotistical
      arrogant
      foolish
      selfish
      cruel.

The list of possibilities mounts
as does my guilt.
Is this illness a form of
retribution for past offenses?
Is my illness the price I
must pay?

Something deep within
me stirs and
answers…no.

There is no answer to
my question —
    Why Me?

This illness did not
happen for any good
reason. There is no
meaning to it in my life.

It is, instead, a
consequence of
        being human.

I cannot search for
logic or justice.
Life is not logical
        or fair.

Life simply is.

As I look back on my
life, I have regrets…
    words I wish I had
        not said.
    things I wish I had
        not done.

But the past cannot be changed.
My feelings of guilt only place a
burden upon my heart.

I have asked for and received
forgiveness from others.
But that is not enough to
remove the pain of my
self-reproach.

What more am I to do?

Is it possible that I must
offer myself the same love,
understanding and compassion
I have received from others?

Can I forgive myself?
Will I forgive myself?

There can be no guilt when
there is forgiveness.
Difficult though it is,
        I offer myself forgiveness.

The burden is lifted.
The guilt is gone.

## REFLECTIONS

Do I believe forgiveness is a choice?

Am I able to accept forgiveness from others?

Will I offer and accept self-forgiveness to remove feelings of guilt?

If I have forgiven myself, how do I feel now?

## DEVOTIONS

Dear God,

My decision to love and follow you
was made when I was a child, for even
then, I was convinced of your mercy and
love. And when I erred as a child, I always
knew a loving God in Heaven would
forgive me. Now, as an adult, I reflect
on my past offenses and feel anguish
over them. In the midst of my despair,
I feel your peace descend on my heart.
Once again, you have forgiven me, and
in doing so, have enabled me to forgive
myself.

Amen.

**...I shall not be at all ashamed, but...with full courage now as always Christ will be honored in my body.**

*Philippians 1:20*

Sad
Humiliated
Angry
Miserable
Embarrassed

My self-sufficiency is waning. I am embarrassed that I need others to help me with everyday tasks.

Waiting for others to
assist me is not easy.
It is not that I am
impatient. Waiting just
reminds me of my
inabilities.

I used to be such a
private person.
I enjoyed my time alone
    to bathe
        groom and
        dress myself.

Those precious moments
are too few now.

So many of the things I used to
do for myself are now being
done to me or for me. If I must accept
this — as part of my illness —
then I must identify what I need
from others to lessen the
        shame I am feeling.

I have made a list of what I need.

If I can receive these things,
I will have within my grasp
what I so
        desperately need…
            self-respect
            and dignity.

Speak to me, not about me when I am
    in your presence.
Enjoy my company. Laugh with me.
Listen to me when I speak with you.
Forgive my anger if I lose patience
    with myself.

Respect my need for privacy.
Enable me to keep my feelings of worth.
Show me your love and compassion.
Place items I need within reach of my hands.
Enter my room after you have knocked.
Cry with me. Sorrow shared brings
    emotional comfort.
Treat me as a valued human being, despite
    my disfigurement or disability.

## REFLECTIONS

What situations bring feelings of shame?

What do I need from others to lessen the shame that I feel?

Do I treat myself with dignity and respect?

## DEVOTIONS

Dear God,

There are no feelings of shame or embarrassment when I speak with you. You remind me that in spite of my limitations, the essence of who I am will never change. My loving commitment to you created who I am. My worth is not measured by what I am able to do. I am worthy because I love you and because I am loved by you.

Amen.

# ADJUSTING TO ENDLESS CHANGES

**God is our refuge and strength, a very present help in trouble.**

*Psalms 46:1*

There have been so many
changes since this disease
entered my body.

Some of
     my abilities have
        changed to inabilities
     my strengths to fears
     my self-assurances
        to self-doubts.

Responding to these changes
is not easy.  In the process of
trying to adjust to this
disease, I have lost so much.

I have lost my independence.
I am no longer self-sufficient.

I have lost my sense of
security.  I have so many
questions about my future.

How will this disease progress?
Who will care for me?
Are my finances adequate to
meet my medical needs?

I have lost my ability to complete
plans. The unfinished projects
remind me of skills I may never
be able to use again.

I have lost my dreams and my hopes. A carefree future filled with travel and comfort is no longer a realistic goal.

I have lost some friends who find it too painful to remain in my life. My illness reminds them of their own
vulnerabilities
to disease.

I have lost aspects of myself
and my identity. My physical
body has changed as
have my abilities.

With this loss of appearance
and loss of function,
I feel a loss
of self.

These losses grieve me,
and I mourn them.

As I confront these losses,
I am in touch with an increasing
sense of losing control.

I feel angry because I have
    lost control over my life.

Without control,
    I feel…
        powerless
        hopeless
        dependent
        ineffective
        helpless
        inadequate.

Hospital stays are most
distressing to me. It is
there that I lose the sense
of who I am.

My identity fades as I take
part in my new role
        of patient.

My thoughts, feelings
and preferences are lost
in the medical regimen I
am told I must follow.

I am given no opportunity to
decide what will be done for me
or when it will occur.
The hospital routines add to
my sense of isolation.
To many of the medical staff,
I am...

> an entity without rights,
> a disease to be treated.

And in response, I feel...
> powerless
> hopeless
> dependent
> ineffective
> helpless
> inadequate.

I feel a loss of control.

Being hospitalized and receiving
treatment helps control my
pain and the progression
        of this disease.

For that, I am grateful.

But the emotional price
I pay is great. It is only when
I return home where I am more
in control of my environment
and myself that I begin to feel
better about
        who I am.

Being home has its own set
of adjustments. It is here
that I interact with loved ones.

Sometimes, the struggle
seems greater for my loved
ones. They share their feelings
of helplessness as they search
for ways to help me adjust
to this disease.

Learning about the illness and the
path of progression to expect
helps us to adjust, for it
lessens some of the
uncertainties that are a
part of the future.

Teaching my loved ones
how to care for me, when
needed, lessens their feelings
of helplessness and provides
them with something
important to do.

I try to impress upon them,
that while their actions
help me, it is
    their loving
        presence
    that heals me.

I don't think I could
cope with this illness
    without feeling
        their love.

There is grief for my loved
ones. They, too, have
lost many things.

They have lost a healthy
person in their life
who was needed for
emotional and
        financial security.

They have lost someone
who was always busy,
maintaining the home,
caring for the children.

They have lost the plans
for retirement years.

They have lost the dreams
for a future where
    illness plays no part.

They have lost the comfort
    of their regular
        daily life routine.

The whole family life situation
is changing. Things I can no
longer do are being
        done by others.

Responsibilities shift,
tasks change, emotions rise.

There is anger and resentment.

Someone feels burdened with
the changes that are occurring.
The stability that once existed
    is now gone.

Home is no longer a refuge
from the outside pressures
of life. Home is now a
source of pressure because
    of my illness.

There is guilt
        because of the anger.

There are questions. How can
anger be justified when a loved
one is ill? But I understand the
frustrations and the emotional
and physical depletion they are
experiencing
        because of my illness.

Anger is okay.
        Guilt is not necessary.

There is sorrow because of
the losses they are experiencing.

There is hopelessness,
     for there may be no cure
     or chance for recovery.

There is a longing to return
     to the world of yesterday
     when there was
               peace
                 comfort
                   stability
                     health.

My illness is not only within
me. The disease spreads to
all my loved ones and causes
them anguish.

I feel I am a burden.

I wish I could change things
so that life would be easier
        for those I love.

I cannot.

Therein lies my deepest sadness.

        I love them so.

## REFLECTIONS

What are some of the adjustments I have had to make because of this illness?

What are the most difficult changes I have had to make?

What has helped me make these changes?

## REFLECTIONS

How is my illness affecting my loved ones?

How can I help them as they try to adjust to my illness?

Has anything remained constant for me or for my loved ones?

## DEVOTIONS

Dear God,

I do not know which is more difficult
for me — adjusting to this illness or seeing
the hardships my loved ones must endure.
I have struggled to ease their burdens, but
my attempts have been in vain. So, I come
to you and place my family in your
outstretched arms, confident that you will
heal their heartache and bring them peace.
Lift them up, dear God, and sustain them,
as you have sustained me throughout my life.

Amen.

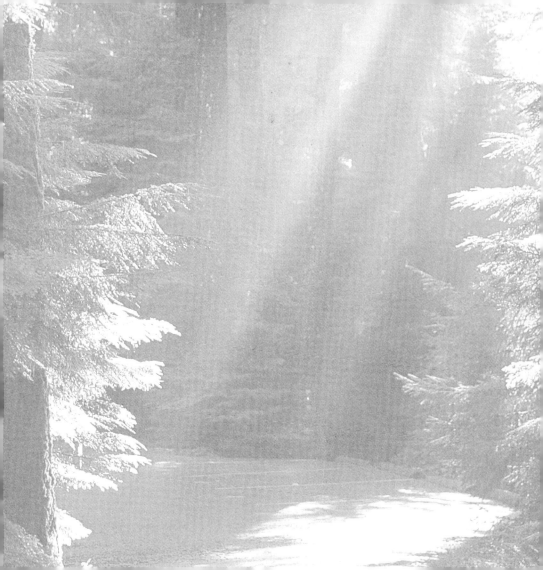

# SURVIVAL

My desire is to depart and be with Christ, for that is far better. But to remain in the flesh is more necessary on your account.

*Philippians 1:23-24*

Life is becoming a
constant struggle.
I exist from day
    to day.
I search for meaning
in my life
    and find none.
There seems to be no
purpose to my existence.

I am not needed
    as I was before.
I cannot perform
    as I did before.
I am beginning to question
    What I am.
        Who I am...

Thoughts of suicide
enter my mind. Is that
action possibly the answer
    to the anguish
        I am feeling?
    to the pain
    I am bringing
        to my loved ones?

Or will my death at
my own hands only
    hurt them more?

Suicide is a choice —
    a release from
      the disease.
    a final farewell
      to life and
        to all that I love.

At times, it seems to
be the logical answer,
    for I feel as though
      I am steadily
        dying.

Why not hasten the
    process?

The choice is mine.

The decision to end
    my life is
        irreversible.

I cannot decide today.
I will see what
    tomorrow brings.

Tomorrow has come.

I feel despondent.
I look in the mirror only
    to see a stranger there.

What has become
        of my life?

What has become
        of me?

I have allowed this disease
to do more than affect me
physically.

I have allowed it to affect
my thoughts,
my feelings,
my reason
for being.

I have allowed it to take
away all meaning
in my life.

If I allow this to continue,
I have no chance
of survival.

Will I choose to live?
The decision must be made,
and it must be made
NOW.



I choose to live.

**REFLECTIONS**

How long have I lived with this illness?

How has this illness affected my thoughts
and my reason for living?

What do I need from myself and from others
to help me choose survival?

## DEVOTIONS

Dear God,

I believe in the preciousness of life.
I have always tried to honor my physical
existence in this world.  But lately, I have
also felt the yearning to return home to you
and to leave this earthly body behind.
Please surround me with your loving
presence, so that I may find a way to
come home to you while I remain
in this world.

Amen.

# HEALING

I have called you by name,
you are mine...You are
precious in my eyes and
honored, and I love you.

*Isaiah 43:1,4*

I choose to live, and
I choose to live
        with meaning
            and
            purpose.

Who am I?

Am I defined
        by my appearance?
        by my abilities?

Do I really want to limit
the meaning of who I am
            to just two aspects
            of myself?

What else makes me
who I am?

What is it about me
that makes me
worthwhile
lovable
special?

I am a combination
of many qualities.

Within me lies –
            sensitivity
            compassion
            gentleness
            kindness
            understanding
            caring
            humor
            love
            joy
            creativity
            wisdom
            affection
            honesty
            fairness
            forgiveness.

These qualities remain
constant in spite
of my disease.

They have always been
a part of me.
Knowing that
gives me inner strength
rekindles my feelings
of worth and
restores a feeling of hope
for the future.

Life takes on a new meaning.

I am beginning to see myself
in a new light.

Facing this crisis has given
me increased
sensitivity and
awareness.
The self-doubts have changed
to renewed confidence.

The inabilities have evolved
into new and
different skills.

The change in my physical
appearance has led to
an awareness of
the beauty that has
always existed
within me.

When this disease first
entered my body, I struggled
to understand the message
    it brought to my life.

Now, I realize it is I
who must decide what
        that message will be.

It is I who must give this
disease a meaning
        in my life.

My reactions to this illness
        determine that meaning.

If I choose to respond with
bitterness and anger,
    then I become
    a bitter and angry person.

If I choose to respond with
    an acceptance of the
    unfairness of my suffering
    and with a determination to
    live fully
        in spite of my illness
        then
        I open my life to
        limitless possibilities
        for new growth.

With this response, I am
able to explore my capacities for —
       strength
       patience
       cheerfulness
       insight
       love
       and becoming
               me.

And I can enhance those
qualities that make me
       special
       worthy
       and
       loved.

Qualities that are me.

Tomorrow is a new day.
A day filled with
opportunities
challenges
hopes and
dreams.

The fear of tomorrow
is gone.
The pain of yesterday
is lessened.

The strength, the love
and the acceptance
of who I am
make today
a more beautiful day.

## REFLECTIONS

Has this illness changed my outlook on life?
If so, in what way?

How will I choose to respond to my illness?
What meaning will I give this illness in my
life?

## REFLECTIONS

What inner qualities have remained a part of
me in spite of this illness?

What makes me a special and worthwhile
person?

**DEVOTIONS**

Dear God,

My devotion to you has spanned my lifetime. Loving you has always brought me joy. Now, I reflect on the realization that you love me. Being loved by you is a truth that humbles me, and at the same time, lifts my spirit to new heights. I am no longer my disease. I am a child of God, loved completely for who I am. In that love, I find consolation and inner peace.

Amen.

# PEACE

**Thou dost keep him in perfect peace whose mind is stayed on Thee, because he trusts in Thee.**

*Isaiah 26:3*

Many days have passed
now, and while my future
remains uncertain, there
exists within me
      a peacefulness
      that enables me
      to live
            meaningfully
            joyously and
            fully.

There are still days
of rain —
      days of physical pain
      and emotional discomfort.

And on those days, I have
learned to look for
      the sun
      within myself
      within others.
For when I do, a rainbow
fills my thoughts,
      giving me the
      inner peace
        and healing
          I need.

I am in a different place now.
I have struggled with this
illness, and I have found
    some answers
        for my life.

I accept life as it is.
I give thanks for the love
    that surrounds me.
I look to the possibilities
    and opportunities
    of each day and
I rejoice with the knowledge
    of who I am.

Therein lies my peace.

## REFLECTIONS

I am a worthwhile, unique and
   beautiful person.
No matter what life brings to me,
   my worth
   my uniqueness and
   my beauty
      will never change.

**DEVOTIONS**

Dear God,

Your love has taught me that inner
peace is not found in my external world.
Instead, it is found where it has always
existed…deep within me. I can find
that place of tranquility by turning my
thoughts to you and resting in the knowledge
that you are always with me.

Amen.

## GOD'S GIFT
## OF HEALING

**For I am convinced that nothing
can ever separate us from God's love.**

*Romans* 8:38

**Lo, I am with you always.**

*Mathew 28:20*

God has been patient with me
during this illness.

When I was angry,
He did not turn away.

When I was filled with despair,
He sent His compassion in the
arms of those who held me.

When I was filled with guilt
and remorse,
He gently whispered His
forgiveness in my heart.

When I was ashamed of the
changes in my body, He reminded
me that I was made in His image
with an inner beauty
that was eternal.

When I was bitter and called
Him unjust and cruel,
He listened and shed
tears in silence.

When my heart was breaking
for my loved ones, He
encompassed them in the circle
of His love and brought them
comfort and strength.

When I found a renewed
      meaning in my life, in spite
      of my illness, He shared my joy.

My path has never been
      traveled alone.
Throughout this experience,
      God has offered the gentle
      warmth of His constant love.

Now, I bask in the glow of
      His love, and I feel the healing
      power of His compassion.
Death is no longer an enemy
      to be feared. It is, instead,
      the final path to my home
                  with God.

My friends and loved ones
     pray for my body to heal.
They do not understand that
     my healed body may take
     the form of
          a resurrected body.

For is not true healing found
     in the glory of the resurrection?

When my time comes to leave
     this earthly home, I hope the
     memories of moments shared
     will help heal the sense of loss
     for my loved ones.

Memories are a gift from
God to those left behind.

They bring comfort, joy
and laughter, and they
enable me to live forever
in the hearts of
those I love.

## REFLECTIONS

Let not your hearts be troubled; believe
in God, believe also in me. In my
Father's house are many rooms;
if it were not so, would I have told
you that I go and prepare a place
for you?...I will come again and
will take you to myself, that where
I am you may be also.

I am the way, the truth, and the life.

*John 14:2-3,6*

## DEVOTIONS

Dear God,

May your love bring peace and
comfort to my loved ones,
and as for me,
may I rest in your arms.

Amen.

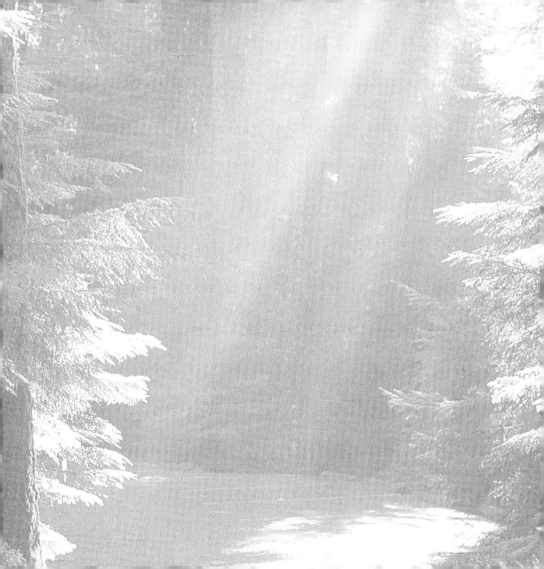

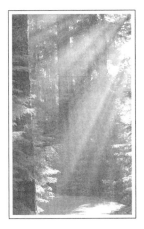

# ABOUT PATIENT PRESS

Patient Press' has a simple mission: "We help people live meaningful lives, despite their illness."

We fulfill this mission by publishing books and other resources to provide practical encouragement for people living with illness. Our Website, www.patientpress.com, offers free information, and includes links to other sites that provide information to help patients make informed decisions.

Our books include:

- *Living Better: Every Patient's Guide to Living with Illness* (ISBN 0-9701545-1-8, $14.95, © 2001) is an empowering, practical resource for the 90 million Americans who live with chronic, life-changing illness. It offers a practical approach to the mind-body-spirit connection and informs, equips, and encourages. Authors Carol Langenfeld, M.S.Ed., M.S.W., and Doug Langenfeld have drawn on their experience as patients to show patients how to take charge of their lives and their health care and live meaningful lives.

- *Living Better: A Christian Group Study Guide* (ISBN 0-9701545-2-6, $6.95, © 2002) is a companion guide for group studies and support groups managing the practical, emotional, and spiritual issues surrounding chronic illness. Each session includes daily Bible readings and questions to generate personal and group reflection and discussion. Experienced patients Carol and Doug Langenfeld draw on their a Christian faith to create this group study guide.

- *Faith and Illness: Reflections on God's Sustaining Love*
(ISBN 0-9701545-3-4, $9.95, © 2002) is a companion for anyone living with illness. It uses heart-touching poetic prose, reflective questions, and prayers, reminding them of God's sustaining compassion and His everlasting love, comfort on days when their hearts are weary from the struggle, and a guide to a fuller understanding of the emotional impact of serious illness. Author Nancy Groves, M.S.W., C.S.W., a medical social worker, has over 20 years experience as a counselor and educator. She has extensive experience conducting seminars and speaking on death and dying issues, including serving on the Michigan Department of Public Health AIDS Advisory Board. She holds Michigan's highest social work credential.

Future projects include *I Can't Get Sick: I've Got Work to Do,* drawing on the experiences of people who have had to make time to be sick to explore the emotional impact of illness, especially when life in the workplace is affected.

Publications are available in bookstores, on-line booksellers, and directly from the publisher:

Patient Press
6475 Perimeter Drive, Box 110
Dublin, Ohio 43016
Phone 614/799-1444
Fax 614/799-1448
www.patientpress.com